# Metabolical Code:

**Processed food's seduction and deception. Nutrition and contemporary medical practice.**

By

*Mark M. Crosley*

*Mark M. Crosley*



I sincerely thank all of the students that shared their stories with me in order to assist me in finishing these, and I am extremely excited to come up with these ideas for metabolic code. It is not a simple task at all. But it is finished today.

# Content

# Introduction

You have probably heard of the terms slow metabolism"
and "fast metabolism" thrown around in online health and
weight loss spaces. But what precisely do those phrases
mean?

Well, slow and quick isn't quite the ideal way to describe
metabolical coding. However, your metabolic health is
still extremely, really important.

In this post, we'll define metabolic code and examine the
ideal foods and diets for metabolic wellness, as well as
the items you should avoid. Let's go!

Metabolical coding, in general, is all about how your
body turns the food you ingest into energy.

When you eat, your blood sugar rises, and the hormone
insulin is created by the pancreas to transfer this sugar
into your cells. Some of this sugar is absorbed instantly as
energy. When there is extra sugar, though, it is deposited
as body fat.

If you're not metabolically healthy, your body may be
insulin resistant; thus, your blood sugar levels stay higher,
and your body releases more insulin to compensate. The
final outcome is higher blood sugar levels and higher
insulin levels.

Insulin resistance generally goes hand-in-hand with
chronic inflammation, which may lead to severe health
problems, like poor heart health.

Cardiometabolic health relates to your metabolic health

and your heart health but is often used interchangeably with the phrase metabolic code.

Metabolic syndrome is a constellation of symptoms that signal poor metabolic health. If you fulfill the criteria for metabolic syndrome, you may be at an elevated risk for heart disease, type 2 diabetes, stroke, some types of cancer, and more.

To be diagnosed with metabolic syndrome, you must meet three of these five criteria[*]:

o A waist of 35+ inches for women or 40+ inches for men
A triglyceride level of at least 150 mg/dL o A low HDL cholesterol level of less than 50 mg/dL for women or less than 40 mg/dL for men
o Blood pressure at or above 130/85 fasting blood sugar of 100 mg/dL or above

Note: These are the standards for metabolic syndrome in the U.S.; however, the criteria in your country may differ significantly.

Any of the characteristics on this list can serve as a hint that your metabolic health may not be optimal. However, if you fulfill the criteria for metabolic syndrome, it's a good idea to start trying to reverse these health issues before they evolve into something more severe.

*Mark M. Crosley*

# Chapter 1

# Nutrition and Dietitians:

In terms of both health and development, nutrition is an essential component. There is a correlation between increased nutrition and improved health in infants, children, and mothers; stronger immune systems; safer pregnancy and childbirth; a lower risk of non-communicable diseases (such as diabetes and cardiovascular disease); and a longer life span.

If children are healthy, they learn better. They are more productive and have the ability to generate possibilities that can progressively break the cycles of poverty and hunger. People who have proper nourishment are more productive.

Every form of malnutrition poses major risks to the health of both humans and other animals. In today's world, the world is confronted with a double burden of malnutrition, which comprises both undernutrition and overweight, particularly in nations with low and moderate standards of living. There are many different types of malnutrition, such as undernutrition (wasting or stunting), insufficient vitamins or minerals, overweight, obesity, and the noncommunicable diseases that are caused by diet-related conditions.

# Expectations Regarding Nutrition That You Have to Unlearn:

There is no such thing as good or terrible food, but there are foods that are superior to others in terms of their nutritional value. But your dichotomous thinking regarding food is setting you up for failure. What you should do instead is incorporate your favorite meals and "fun stuff" into your diet. This will make your diet more sustainable, and as a result, you will be more likely to adhere to it and achieve your goals.

2. No food group in isolation will lead you to store fat. Carbs and fats do not make you fat. Too many calories lead people to gain weight.

3. You don't have to starve yourself to lose weight. Just ask yourself this. How many times have you restricted eating to reduce weight? How long did it last for? And was it enjoyable? - I seriously doubt it.

4. Cheat days are not a genuine thing; if you need to cheat on your diet, you're not doing it right. As above, include your favorite meals and fun stuff in your everyday diet, and you don't need to cheat.

5. Everyone's calories are different; do not imitate anyone else's calories.

6. You don't have to watch calories, but calories are important and will ultimately represent your body

weight.

7. Consistency is vital, not perfection. No one can be perfect with their diet. You are going to have good and bad days, but your all-or-nothing mentality is forcing you to give up at the drop of a hat and finish back in the same cycle you were in six months ago.

## Dietitians

Dietitians enable people to improve their health by offering expert nutrition and dietary guidance. A dietician can help you manage health concerns, such as:

1. diabetes;

2. eating disorders.
3. Heart disease
4. Obesity

Dietitians understand how nutrition impacts the body and apply this information when treating you. Using the latest scientific information, dietitians partner with you to build a specific plan to match your needs.

# Chapter 2

# What is considered to be healthy?

Being "healthy" may mean so many different things to different people. Believe it or not, it's not solely related to physical beauty, although many people are quick to assume that it is. "Skinny" doesn't necessarily imply you're healthy, and in the same breath, a high BMI doesn't necessarily equate to an unhealthy individual. There are a lot of aspects that go into the evaluation of whether you are genuinely living a healthy life. Whether it's the food you consume, the amount of physical activity in your routine, or the social activities you engage in, it all connects together. According to the World Health Organization (WHO), the word health means "a state of complete physical, mental, and social well-being," and this involves the use of personal and social resources to guarantee that an individual can function throughout their everyday life. In other words, if your body can efficiently manage threats to your system (physically, psychologically, or emotionally), you are deemed to be healthy. Keep in mind that health care experts are skilled individuals that are qualified to analyze every element of your health, but there are certain broad symptoms that suggest that you are in excellent condition from a physical and mental perspective:


1. You are eating a diet that is well-rounded and includes lots of whole foods. No one is perfect, but the key is trying your best to integrate whole foods and optimal nutrients into your daily diet as consistently as possible. That involves integrating full, unadulterated foods into your meals. Occasionally overspending is good, but it is absolutely not suggested regularly! It's all about balance.

2. You can skillfully manage a broad spectrum of emotions. Too frequently, people think you have to be happy all the time. That is far from the truth. Happiness seems substantially more healthy when you feel a range of emotions in between those pleasant times. The trick is properly implementing ways to manage those not-so-great sensations and circumstances. If you discover that, more frequently than not, you are struggling to manage your tension, anger, or anxiety about things, there may be a need to get help with that. A true measure of healthy emotional well-being is the ability to welcome and manage a range of emotions, recognizing they are not permanent.

3. You have enough energy to get through your day and

complete your daily to-do list. Whether we are talking about physical energy or mental energy, having the ability to focus and do the tasks you want to do each day is a sign of good health. If you are struggling to go through tasks you regularly do in a day, this could be an indication of concern connected to your health. It could be as simple as clocking more quality hours of sleep at night or eating more of the proper meals.

4. You feel refreshed when you get up. If you're hitting the pillow at night and you wake up feeling like you hardly slept, there's a concern there. The appropriate quantity of sleep is not only crucial for your body but for your intellect as well. Getting eight hours of sleep is preferable but not always possible for everyone, which is why quality sleep is just as vital. The CDC finds that more than a third of adults in the country indicate they are not getting enough sleep.

5. You add moderate exercise and movement to your everyday routine. The recommended amount of exercise for optimal health is 150 weekly minutes of moderate activity, like brisk walking. You can easily satisfy this expectation without having to acquire a membership to a local gym. Especially with the great weather we're currently experiencing, hopping on a bike, traveling to the pool for a swim, or taking a walk around the block would be the perfect way to soak up

some vitamin D while getting in some exercise! Depending on your degree of physical fitness, it is always vital to contact a professional who can guide you on the correct activities to engage in.

6. When thinking about your overall health, it is crucial to realize that it is all about establishing a healthy balance between your mental and physical fitness. Even if you believe you "don't need help" in certain areas, there are always proactive measures to preserve your present level of health and prepare yourself for unanticipated issues in the future. At Heyl Family Practice, for example, there are physicians to help manage your physical health needs, such as an annual physical, and counselors to manage your mental health needs. Together, these professionals can help us design an ideal and comprehensive health plan for our patients.

7. Regardless, being healthy looks different from person to person. If you make an attempt to engage in proactive health and wellness activities and routines, including maintenance of ongoing conditions and preventative treatment, you are taking the appropriate measures. The key is consistency, listening to your body, and taking action when you see or feel something troubling. If you haven't scheduled your yearly physical yet, today is the perfect time to do it! We'd love to see you and check on the status of your health and wellness.

# Chapter 3

# What is healthy food for older children and teenagers?

Healthy cuisine for pre-teen and teenage children contains a wide variety of fresh foods from the five food groups:
1. vegetables
2. fruit
3. grain foods
4. reduced-fat dairy or dairy-free alternatives
5. protein.
Each food category offers distinct nutrients, which your child's body needs to grow and perform properly.
That's why we need to eat a mix of foods from all five food categories.

# Fruit and vegetables:

Fruit and vegetables give your youngster energy, vitamins, antioxidants, fiber, and hydration. These nutrients can protect your child against problems later in life, including conditions like heart disease, stroke, and several malignancies.

Encourage your youngster to choose fruit and vegetables at every meal and for snacks. This contains fruit and vegetables of diverse colors, textures, and flavors, both fresh and cooked.

Wash fruit to eliminate dirt or pesticides, and leave any edible skin on because the skin provides nutrients too. Some teenagers don't like eating a lot of fruit and vegetables. You may help by being a healthy eating role model. If your child sees you eating a wide selection of veggies and fruit, they are more inclined to try them too. And you can encourage your youngster to make healthy choices by offering plenty of fruit and vegetables in your family's meals and snacks.

# Grain foods:

Grain foods include bread, pasta, noodles, breakfast cereals, couscous, rice, corn, quinoa, polenta, oats, and barley. These foods give your child the energy they need to grow, develop, and learn.

Grain meals with a low glycaemic index, including wholegrain pasta and breads, will give your child longer-lasting energy and keep them feeling fuller for longer.

Reduced-fat dairy foods and dairy-free alternatives

Key dairy foods are milk, cheese, and yogurt. These foods are good providers of calcium and protein.

In puberty, your child needs additional calcium to help them reach peak bone mass and build strong bones for life. So urge your child to have different forms of dairy each day—for example, glasses of milk, cheese pieces, bowls of yogurt, and so on.

If your child doesn't consume dairy, it's crucial for them to eat dairy-free foods that are rich in calcium— for example, tofu, kale, bok choy, almonds, seeds, tinned fish with bones, and calcium-fortified foods like cereal, soy milk, and bread. Not all dairy replacements are fortified with calcium, though, so make sure to read food labels.

## Protein:

Protein-rich foods include lean meat, fish, chicken, eggs, beans, lentils, chickpeas, tofu, and almonds. These nutrients are vital for your child's growth and muscle development, especially during puberty.

These protein-rich foods also offer additional vitamins and minerals like iron and omega-3 fatty acids, which are particularly necessary during adolescence.

Healthy drinks for teenagers

Water is the healthiest drink for your child. It's also the cheapest. Most tap water is treated with fluoride for strong teeth, too.

Reduced-fat milk is also a good drink option for teenagers. It's high in calcium, which is helpful for bone formation.

Foods and drinks to limit

Encourage your child to restrict the amount of 'sometimes' food they eat. This means your child will have more room for nutritious, daily foods.

'Sometimes' foods include fast food, takeout, and junk food such as hot chips, potato chips, dim sims, pies, burgers, and takeaway pizza. They also include cakes, chocolate, sweets, cookies, doughnuts, and pastries. These foods can be heavy in salt, saturated fat, and sugar and lacking in fiber. If teenagers routinely eat certain items, it can increase their risk of teenage overweight and obesity and associated health issues like type 2 diabetes.

Your youngster should restrict sugary liquids, including fruit juice, cordials, sports drinks, flavored waters, soft drinks, and flavored milks. Sweet drinks are high in sugar and lacking in nutrition.

Too many sweet drinks can contribute to unhealthy

weight gain, obesity, and tooth disease. These drinks fill your child up and can make them less eager for healthier meals.

Foods and drinks with caffeine aren't recommended for older children and teenagers because caffeine can impact how much calcium the body can absorb. Caffeine is also a stimulant, which means it offers youngsters false energy. Too much caffeine might create sleep problems as well as problems concentrating at school.

Foods and drinks with caffeine include coffee, tea, energy drinks, and chocolate.

# Chapter 4

## What should adults eat:

Eating a healthy, balanced diet is a crucial element of maintaining excellent health and can help you feel your best.

This includes eating a wide variety of foods in the proper proportions and consuming the right amount of food and drink to achieve and maintain a healthy body weight.

This page includes healthy eating guidelines for the general population.

People with unique dietary needs or a medical condition

should seek their doctor or a qualified dietician for help.

Food groups in your diet

The Eatwell Guide shows that to have a healthy, balanced diet, people should attempt to:

1. Eat at least 5 pieces of a variety of fruit and veggies every day.
2. base meals on higher-fiber starchy foods like potatoes, bread, rice, or pasta.
3. have some dairy or dairy alternatives (such as soy drinks).
4. Eat some beans, grains, fish, eggs, meat, and other protein.
5. Choose unsaturated oils and spreads and eat them in small amounts.
6. Drink enough water (at least 6 to 8 glasses a day).

If you're having foods and drinks that are heavy in fat, salt, and sugar, consume them less often and in small amounts.

Try to choose a variety of different foods from the five main food groups to acquire a wide range of nutrients.

Most individuals in the UK consume and drink too many calories, too much saturated fat, sugar, and salt, and not enough fruit, vegetables, oily fish, or fiber.

The Eatwell Guide does not apply to children under the age of 2 because they have distinct nutritional demands. Between the ages of 2 and 5 years, children should gradually migrate to eating the same foods as the rest of the family in the amounts specified in the Eatwell

Guide. Fruit and vegetables: are you getting your 5 A Day?

Fruit and vegetables are a wonderful source of vitamins, minerals, and fiber and should make up just over a third of the food you eat each day.

It's advised that you consume at least five servings of a variety of fruit and vegetables every day. They can be fresh, frozen, tinned, dried, or juiced.

There's evidence that those who consume at least 5 servings of fruit and vegetables a day have a lower risk of heart disease, stroke, and several other malignancies. Eating five pieces is not as hard as it sounds.

A chunk is:

1. 80g of fresh, tinned, or frozen fruit and vegetables
2. 30g of dry fruit, which should be confined to mealtimes
3. 150 ml glass of fruit juice or smoothie, but do not consume more than 1 portion a day as these drinks are sweet and can harm teeth.

Just 1 apple, banana, pear, or similar-sized fruit equals 1 piece each.

A piece of pineapple or melon is likewise one part, and three heaping tablespoons of veggies are another portion.

Adding a spoonful of dried fruit, such as raisins, to your morning cereal is an easy way to achieve one portion. You could also replace your mid-morning biscuit for a banana and add a side salad to your meal.

In the evening, enjoy a dish of vegetables with dinner and fresh fruit with plain, lower-fat yogurt for dessert to reach your 5 A Day.

# Chapter 5

# Food classification:

Foods are classified on the basis of their actions:
Energy-giving foods
The carbs, lipids, and protein are classified as calorie nutrients so that the body can accomplish the necessary duties. Rice, chapatti, bread, potatoes, sugar, oil, butter, and ghee are examples of energy-boosting foods.
Body-building foods

Foods such as proteins, lipids, and carbs are also termed body-building foods. They are the nutrients that make bodily tissues. Fish, pork, poultry, eggs, legumes, nuts, and milk are some body-building foods.

Protective foods

Vitamins and minerals are the nutrients that serve to control biological processes. They protect us from many ailments. Fruits and vegetables are some examples. Therefore, we must eat these regularly. amounts necessary for cells and organisms are classified as macronutrients: Macronutrients are required in substantial quantities daily. Proteins, carbs, and lipids are macronutrients. They are the backbone of any diet.

Micronutrients: Micronutrients are needed in small quantities (typically in levels less than milligrams). These nutrients are involved in controlling metabolism and energy activities. They are vitamins and minerals.

# Food addiction:

For men and women suffering from an addiction to food, highly palatable foods (which are often rich in fat, sugar, and/or salt) elicit chemical reactions in the brain that generate feelings of pleasure and satisfaction. This reaction has been interpreted as akin to an addict's response to their substance of choice, as it activates the same brain reward center.

Food addicts become hooked upon the "good" feelings that are gained from consuming particular meals, which typically creates a continual urge to eat, even when not hungry. These practices form a vicious loop. As the food addict continues to binge on foods that create happy feelings, they often overindulge and consume more than is required for satisfaction and adequate nutrition.
This can lead to various physical, mental, and social problems, such as digestive disorders, heart disease, obesity, low self-worth, despair, and loneliness. A food addict will often re-engage in these damaging habits, even with undesired outcomes, due to the need for induced emotions of pleasure.

## Eating healthily for your waistline and wallet:

1. Cooking makes cents.
The first tip for saving is to cook your own food—for all meals—rather than eating at restaurants (particularly fast-food establishments). Self-prepared meals are nearly always significantly less expensive, and for added convenience, try making larger portions so you can make meals from leftovers later in the week.
• Another method to extend your budget? Look into food coops in your area; being a member may help you access healthier goods at a lesser price.
2. Minimize meat.

Plant-based diets are not only regarded as best for health; they also tend to be more inexpensive. Animal proteins normally cost more, so rather than create a meal around meat, vary things up. Pick a veggie for your primary meal, and include meat sparingly. You'll still get to experience both, but in a proportion that is healthier for you and your budget.

• An additional advantage? Plant-based goods like nuts and healthy grains have a longer shelf life than meat, which tends to perish more quickly.

3. Spend more attention, spend less money.

When eating thoughtfully, many people find they are satisfied with less food. Eating less, in turn, can translate into buying less. So while mindfulness is wonderful for health, it has an extra budget benefit, too.

In a meta-analysis (2) of 24 studies about the effect of food intake memory and awareness on eating, data suggested that attentive eating is likely to influence food intake.

• Eating when distracted produced a slight increase in immediate intake but raised subsequent intake even more.

• The more you pay attention, the less you eat—both at that time and afterward.

Practice eating consciously, and check if minimizing distractions saves you money.

4. The contradiction of processed

Fats, such as nuts, and protein sources, like fish and chicken, tend to cost more, but oftentimes you can be happy eating less of these "higher quality" items. A simpler way to express it is that the higher the quality, the less it takes to fulfill your appetite. Fats and proteins tend to be more satiating, so it takes less of them to feel full. • Highly processed foods, on the other hand, tend to make you hungrier. Typically full of sugar and refined carbohydrates, highly refined meals like cereals, cakes, cookies, and chips cause your blood sugar to soar and subsequently plummet, resulting in increased appetite even after you've eaten.

So be wise when picking what to consume. A bag of nuts may appear pricy, but it may easily last a week or more. A bag of chips can have a lower price, but it could be gone in one hour! Processed foods may appear to be less expensive, but you'll likely eat them faster—and eat more of them.

5. Examine how you compute costs.

Most people conceive of food expenses as simply the amount they pay at the grocery store. However, it's a more complex equation. The cost of your food isn't determined at the checkout line; the real cost of your food is estimated much later, when you examine its influence on your health. Paying extra now may save you money later on health care costs.

## Final summary

Healthy eating has several benefits, such as reducing the

*Mark M. Crosley*

risk of heart disease, stroke, obesity, and type 2 diabetes. A person may also increase their mood and acquire more energy by maintaining a balanced diet.

www.ingramcontent.com/pod-product-compliance
Lightning Source LLC
Chambersburg PA
CBHW071052260726

48660CB00008B/3186